Table of Contents

Osteoporosis is a bone disease that develops when bone mineral density and bone mass decreases, or when the quality or structure of bone changes. This can lead to a decrease in bone strength that can increase the risk of fractures (broken bones).

Osteoporosis is a "silent" disease because you typically do not have symptoms, and you may not even know you have the disease until you break a bone. Osteoporosis is the major cause of fractures in postmenopausal women and in older men. Fractures can occur in any bone but happen most often in bones of the hip, vertebrae in the spine, and wrist.

However, you can take steps to help prevent the disease and fractures by:

Staying physically active by participating in weight-bearing exercises such as walking.

Drinking alcohol in moderation.

Quitting smoking, or not starting if you don't smoke.

Taking your medications, if prescribed, which can help prevent fractures in people who have osteoporosis.

Eating a nutritious diet rich in calcium and vitamin D to help maintain good bone health.

BREAKFAST

1. Brown Rice

Prep Time: 5 Minutes

Cook Time: 10 Minutes

Servings: 1

Ingredients

- 1 cup spinach
- 2 tbsp carrot grated
- 2 cups brown rice
- 1 egg
- 2 tbsp cheese grated
- 2.5 ounces avocado (half an avocado)
- 1 tbsp olive oil extra virgin
- 1/2 cup blueberries
- 1 tbsp sesame seeds
- 1 tsp pesto to top
- 1/2 fresh squeezed lemon

Instructions

1. Start by prepping your ingredients!

2. Cook your brown rice as per package instructions.

3. Place your egg in a pot and add cold water until the whole egg is covered and there's an additional 1 inch of water on top. Bring to a boil over medium-high heat, then cover. Remove from heat and set aside for 8 to 10 minutes. Drain and place in a bowl of cold water to cool. Once cool, you can peel your egg.

4. Wash all your fruits and veggies. Grate your carrots and cheese, and slice your avocado.

5. Once all your ingredients are prepped, it's time to assemble your bowl. Start by placing your rice at the bottom of the bowl. Then, make it look pretty by arranging the rest of your ingredients separately on top— like I do in the video!

6. Squeeze half a lemon over your bowl and finish with a drizzle of olive oil!

Prep Time: 8 Minutes

Cook Time: 8hrs 2 Minutes

Servings: 1

Ingredients

- ½ cup of rolled oats
- ½ cup of milk
- ½ cup of greek yoghurt
- 1 banana
- 3 fresh dates - sliced
- 1 tablespoon of walnuts - toasted
- 1 teaspoon of chia seeds

Instructions

1. Cut the banana in half and mash in a small bowl before adding the milk, greek yoghurt, 2 of the sliced dates and chia seeds.

2. Mix to combine all of the ingredients before covering the bowl and placing it into the fridge and leaving overnight.

3. The next morning, warm your oats in the microwave for 30 seconds (optional), before slicing the remaining half of the banana and adding it along with the toasted walnuts and remaining sliced date to your oats

Prep Time: 20 Minutes

Cook Time: 40 Minutes

Servings: 6

Ingredients

- 1 kilogram chicken mince
- 1 zucchini 120 grams
- 2 carrots 120 grams
- 50 grams parmesan cheese finely grated
- 2 garlic cloves
- 2 tablespoons mixed herbs
- 2 tablespoons onion flakes
- ½ cup breadcrumbs
- salt and pepper to taste
- Sauce Ingredients
- 700 grams passata
- 140 grams tomato paste
- 200 grams water
- 1 tablespoon mixed herbs
- 1 tablespoon onion flakes
- ½ cup mozzarella

Instructions

1. Preheat your oven to 180 degrees celsius (fan-forced) and lightly grease a large baking dish.

2. In a large bowl, combine the chicken mince, grated zucchini and carrot, parmesan cheese, crushed garlic cloves, 2 tablespoons of mixed herbs, 2 tablespoons of onion flakes, ½ cup of breadcrumbs and add a pinch of salt and pepper to taste.

3. Use a dessertspoon to scoop up the mixture and roll into 24 even sized balls and place into your greased baking dish.

4. Pop the baking dish into your preheated oven and cook for 10 minutes.

5. While the Chicken Parma Balls are cooking, combine the pasta, tomato paste, water, 1 tablespoon of mixed herbs and 1 tablespoon of onion flakes into a medium saucepan and cook over a medium /low heat until the sauce begins to simmer.

6. Remove the Chicken Parma Balls from the oven and carefully pour the tomato sauce over the top.

7. Sprinkle the mozzarella cheese over the top of the sauce and put the Chicken and Vegetable Parma Balls back into the oven to cook for a further 25 minutes or until

the cheese is golden and the chicken has cooked through.

Prep Time: 15 Minutes

Cook Time: 20 Minutes

Servings: 6

Ingredients

- 30 grams butter
- 1 brown onion
- 2 cloves garlic
- 500 grams chicken breast or thigh
- ½ teaspoon ground ginger
- ½ teaspoon cinnamon
- ½ tsp tumeric
- ½ teaspoon cumin
- ½ teaspoon paprika
- 1 teaspoon garam marsala powder
- 100 grams tomato paste
- 400 grams coconut cream
- ¾ cup long grain rice

Instructions

1. Finely chop the onion and crush garlic and add it along with the butter to a large saucepan over a medium heat. Saute for 5 minutes and stir gently until the onion is translucent.

2. Add the chopped chicken pieces (which have been cut into cubes no bigger than 3cm) and all of the spices and cook for 5 minutes, stirring regularly.

3. Add the tomato paste and coconut cream and stir through. Cook for 5 minutes before reducing the heat to medium/low and pop the lid on and cook for a further 5 minutes or until the chicken is cooked through.

4. In the meantime you can cook the rice as per the packed instructions.

5. Serve the Butter Chicken and Rice together.

6. Thermomix Instructions

7. Place the onion (cut in half) and the garlic cloves into your Thermomix bowl and mix for 6 seconds, speed 6.

8. Scrape down the sides of your Thermomix bowl and add the butter, cook for 3 minutes, 100 degrees, speed 1.

9. Scrape down the sides of the Thermomix bowl and add the chicken pieces, ground ginger, cinnamon, tumeric,

cumin, paprika and garam marsala powder. Mix for 6 seconds, speed 2 on REVERSE.

10. Scrape down the sides of the Thermomix bowl and cook for 6 minutes, 100 degrees, speed 1 on REVERSE.

11. In the meantime you can cook the rice as per the packed instructions.

12. Add the tomato paste and coconut cream into your Thermomix bowl and cook for a further 8 minutes, 90 degrees, speed 1, REVERSE.

13. Serve the Butter Chicken and Rice together.

Prep Time: 15 Minutes

Cook Time: 20 Minutes

Servings: 23

Ingredients

- 500 grams chicken mince
- ½ cup breadcrumbs approximately 2 slices of bread
- ½ cup grated zucchini 60 grams
- ½ cup grated parmesan cheese 50 grams
- 2 cloves garlic crushed
- ½ tablespoon onion flakes
- 1 tablespoon tomato relish
- Pinch of salt and pepper

Instructions

1. Preheat your oven to 220 degrees celsius (fan-forced) and lightly grease a non stick baking tray.
2. Place all of the ingredients into a large bowl and mix well to combine.

3. Use a tablespoon to scoop up the chicken mixture and shape into balls. If you find the mixture is still a little 'wet' you can add some more breadcrumbs to help it 'stick' together and shape into balls.

4. Place the chicken balls onto your prepared baking tray and cook for 16 – 18 minutes or until they begin to turn golden and are cooked through when tested.

Prep Time: 20 Minutes

Cook Time: 25 Minutes

Servings: 23

Ingredients

- 500 grams chicken mince see notes
- 1 tablespoon onion flakes optional
- ½ teaspoon salt
- ¼ teaspoon pepper
- 1 cup panko breadcrumbs
- 100 grams parmesan cheese finely grated
- 2 tablespoon dried mixed herbs
- 3 eggs
- olive oil spray

Instructions

1. Preheat your oven to 190 degrees celsius (fan-forced) set aside two non stick baking trays until needed.
2. Place the chicken mince, a pinch of salt and pepper and one egg into a large bowl and mix to combine. Use a

dessert spoon to scoop up the mixture and shape/roll into a nugget shape. Place onto a plate and pop into the fridge until needed.

3. Lightly beat the eggs and place them into a bowl – set aside until needed.

4. Place the panko breadcrumbs, finely grated parmesan cheese and mixed herbs into a bowl and stir to combine.

5. Remove the chicken from the fridge and coat in the egg before transferring to the bowl with the breadcrumb mixture and turn to coat before placing on a baking tray – repeat until all of the mixture has been used.

6. Lightly spray the nuggets with olive oil (optional) before placing them into the oven to cook for 25 minutes or until golden and cooked through.

Prep Time: 10 Minutes

Cook Time: 2hrs 5 Minutes

Servings: 20

Ingredients

- 75 grams butter
- 200 grams white marshmallows
- 6 cups rice bubbles or similar
- 100s & 1000s to decorate optional

Instructions

1. To begin, line the base and sides of a 20 cm cake tin with baking paper - making sure you leave the paper hanging over the edges.
2. In a large bowl, add the rice bubbles and set aside until needed.
3. Place the butter and marshmallows in a small saucepan and cook over a medium heat stirring occasionally until they have both melted and combined.

4. Pour the melted mixture quickly into the bowl with the rice bubbles, and mix until combined.

5. Pour the combined mixture into a slice tin and use a metal spoon to spread across the tin and push down.

6. Sprinkle 100s and 1000s over the top (optional) and place in the fridge for two hours or until set.

7. Once set, remove the slice from the fridge and cut into small squares.

Prep Time: 20 Minutes

Cook Time: 45 Minutes

Servings: 10

Ingredients

- 500 grams beef mince
- 1 carrot
- 1 zucchini
- 1 brown onion
- 1 clove garlic crushed
- 1 teaspoon Worcestershire sauce
- 2 teaspoon soy sauce
- 1 egg
- 2 tablespoon tomato relish or sauce

Instructions

1. Grate the carrot, zucchini and brown onion and place into a large bowl
2. Crush the garlic cloves and add to the bowl.

3. Add the remaining ingredients and using either your hands or a large metal spoon, break up the mince and mix together until combined.

Prep Time: 15 Minutes

Cook Time: 8hrs 5 Minutes

Servings: 10

Ingredients

- 600 g Gravy Beef which has been cut into large pieces.
- 1 tablespoon olive oil
- 1 brown onion - chopped
- 2 celery sticks - chopped
- 1 large carrot - chopped
- 3 cloves of garlic - crushed
- 4 bacon rashers - roughly chopped
- ⅓ cup plain flour
- 400 g can Italian diced tomatoes
- pinch of salt and pepper
- 1 liter of beef stock
- 2 tablespoon of dried mixed herbs
- ½ cup of frozen peas

Instructions

1. Add the olive oil to a large frying pan and add the diced gravy beef. Cook for 3 - 4 minutes until brown on the outside before transferring to your slow cooker.

2. Add the chopped bacon, onion, carrot, celery and crushed garlic to your frying pan and cook for approximately 4 minutes or until the onion begins to turn translucent. Add the plain flour and toss the ingredient to coat and cooking for a further 2 minutes before transferring all of the ingredient (plus any pan juices) to your slow cooker.

3. Add the beef stock, crushed tomatoes and mix herbs and gently stir through before cooking on a slow setting for 8 hours.

4. When there is around half an hour cooking time remaining, add the frozen peas and stir through.

Prep Time: 25 Minutes

Cook Time: 7hrs 5 Minutes

Servings: 4

Ingredients

- 1 tablespoon of olive oil
- 1 kg of chuck or skirt steak cut into 3cm cubes
- 2 carrots
- 2 brown onions
- 2 garlic cloves - crushed
- 2 tablespoons of curry powder
- 600 g of potatoes
- 500 of pumpkin
- 2 x 400g tins of crushed tomatoes
- 1 cup of beef stock
- Salt and Pepper to taste
- 1 cup of frozen baby peas

Instructions

1. Cut the potatoes and pumpkin into approximately 4cm chunks and thickly cut the carrots until they are approximately 2cm thick. Set aside until needed.

2. Heat the olive oil over a medium/high heat in a large frying pan and add the crushed garlic, curry powder, brown onion (which has been cut into quarters) and the beef pieces and cook until the meat in batches until it is just starting to brown.

3. Transfer the contents of the frying pan to your slow cooker and add the chopped potatoes, carrots and pumpkin pieces along with the two tins of crushed tomatoes and beef stock. Cook on the low setting for 7 hours.

4. After approximately 7 hours cooking time, add the frozen peas and stir through. Cook for a further 5 - 10 minutes or until the peas are cooked.

5. Serve this slow cooker Curried Beef and Vegetables with rice or pasta.

Prep Time: 25 Minutes

Cook Time: 1hrs 5 Minutes

Servings: 6

Ingredients

- 2 tablespoons extra-virgin olive oil
- 8 ounces sliced fresh mixed wild mushrooms such as cremini, shiitake, button and/or oyster mushrooms
- 1 ½ cups thinly sliced sweet onion
- 1 tablespoon thinly sliced garlic
- 5 ounces fresh baby spinach (about 8 cups), coarsely chopped
- 6 large eggs
- ¼ cup whole milk
- ¼ cup half-and-half
- 1 tablespoon Dijon mustard
- 1 tablespoon fresh thyme leaves, plus more for garnish
- ¼ teaspoon salt
- ¼ teaspoon ground pepper

- 1 ½ cups shredded Gruyere cheese

Instructions

1. Preheat oven to 375 degrees F. Coat a 9-inch pie pan with cooking spray; set aside.
2. Heat oil in a large nonstick skillet over medium-high heat; swirl to coat the pan. Add mushrooms; cook, stirring occasionally, until browned and tender, about 8 minutes. Add onion and garlic; cook, stirring often, until softened and tender, about 5 minutes. Add spinach; cook, tossing constantly, until wilted, 1 to 2 minutes. Remove from heat.
3. Whisk eggs, milk, half-and-half, mustard, thyme, salt and pepper in a medium bowl. Fold in the mushroom mixture and cheese. Spoon into the prepared pie pan. Bake until set and golden brown, about 30 minutes. Let stand for 10 minutes; slice. Garnish with thyme and serve.

Prep Time: 5 Minutes

Cook Time: 8hrs 5 Minutes

Servings: 5

Ingredients

- 2 1/2 cups old-fashioned rolled oats (see Tip)
- 2 1/2 cups unsweetened nondairy milk, such as almond or coconut
- 6 teaspoons light brown sugar
- 1 ½ teaspoons vanilla extract
- 1 ¼ teaspoons ground cinnamon
- ½ teaspoon salt

Instructions

1. Stir oats, milk, brown sugar, vanilla, cinnamon and salt together in a large bowl. Divide among five 8-ounce jars. Screw on lids and refrigerate overnight or for up to 5 days.

Prep Time: 20 Minutes

Cook Time: 20 Minutes

Servings: 4

Ingredients

- 1 ½ tablespoons extra-virgin olive oil
- ½ cup panko breadcrumbs, preferably whole-wheat
- 1 small clove garlic, minced
- 8 tablespoons grated Parmesan cheese, divided
- 3 tablespoons finely chopped fresh parsley
- 3 large egg yolks
- 1 large egg
- ½ teaspoon ground pepper
- ¼ teaspoon salt
- 1 (9 ounce) package fresh tagliatelle or linguine
- 8 cups baby spinach
- 1 cup peas (fresh or frozen)

Instructions

1. Put 10 cups of water in a large pot and bring to a boil over high heat.
2. Meanwhile, heat oil in a large skillet over medium-high heat. Add breadcrumbs and garlic; cook, stirring frequently, until toasted, about 2 minutes. Transfer to a small bowl and stir in 2 tablespoons Parmesan and parsley. Set aside.
3. Whisk the remaining 6 tablespoons Parmesan, egg yolks, egg, pepper and salt in a medium bowl.
4. Cook pasta in the boiling water, stirring occasionally, for 1 minute. Add spinach and peas and cook until the pasta is tender, about 1 minute more. Reserve 1/4 cup of the cooking water. Drain and place in a large bowl.
5. Slowly whisk the reserved cooking water into the egg mixture. Gradually add the mixture to the pasta, tossing with tongs to combine. Serve topped with the reserved breadcrumb mixture.

Prep Time: 20 Minutes

Cook Time: 30 Minutes

Servings: 8

Ingredients

- 1 tablespoon canola oil
- 1 ½ pounds boneless, skinless chicken breasts, trimmed and cut into bite-size pieces
- 1 small onion, finely chopped
- ⅓ cup all-purpose flour
- 4 cups reduced-fat milk
- 3 cups broccoli florets
- 2 tablespoons water
- 2 (9 ounce) packages precooked brown rice
- 1 ½ cups shredded reduced-fat sharp Cheddar cheese
- 1 teaspoon dry mustard
- ½ teaspoon garlic powder
- ¾ teaspoon salt
- ½ teaspoon ground pepper
- 1 cup prepared crispy fried onions

Instructions

1. Preheat oven to 400°F.

2. Heat oil in a large high-sided ovenproof skillet over medium-high heat. Add chicken and chopped onion; cook, stirring occasionally, until the chicken is no longer pink on the outside, about 7 minutes. Sprinkle the mixture with flour and cook, stirring occasionally, for 1 minute. Add milk to the pan and bring to a boil, stirring frequently. (Be careful, the pan will be very full.) Boil, stirring, for 1 minute.

3. Meanwhile, place broccoli and water in a microwave-safe container. Cover and microwave on High until the broccoli is tender, about 3 minutes. Drain.

4. Remove the pan from the heat and carefully stir in rice, cheese, dry mustard, garlic powder, salt, pepper and the broccoli. Sprinkle with crispy onions.

5. Bake the casserole until bubbling at the edges, about 10 minutes. Let stand for 5 minutes before serving.

Prep Time: 35 Minutes

Cook Time: 1hr 10 Minutes

Servings: 4

Ingredients

- 2 tablespoons extra-virgin olive oil
- 1 medium onion, chopped
- 1 poblano pepper, seeded and chopped
- ¼ teaspoon salt
- 12 ounces cooked chicken breast, shredded (about 3 cups)
- 1 cup shredded Mexican-blend cheese, divided
- 1 (15 ounce) can enchilada sauce (1 1/2 cups), divided
- 3 medium zucchini (about 1 pound), trimmed
- ⅓ cup sour cream
- 3 tablespoons reduced-fat milk
- 1 cup shredded romaine lettuce
- ½ cup chopped fresh cilantro

Instructions

1. Preheat oven to 425 degrees F. Heat oil in a large skillet over medium-high heat. Add onion, poblano and salt. Cook, stirring frequently, until the vegetables have softened and are beginning to brown, about 6 minutes. Reduce heat to medium if vegetables start to burn. Transfer to a large bowl. Add chicken, 1/2 cup cheese and 1/2 cup enchilada sauce. Stir to combine; set aside.

2. Using a vegetable peeler or mandolin slicer, slice zucchini lengthwise into thin strips Discard any uneven and broken pieces. You should end up with 48 slices.

3. Spread 1/4 cup enchilada sauce on the bottom of a 9-by-13-inch baking dish. Lay three strips of zucchini on a clean work surface, overlapping the edges by 1/4 inch or so. Place 2 generous tablespoons of the chicken filling across the middle of the zucchini strips. Gently roll the zucchini strips around the filling and place seam-side down in the prepared dish. Repeat with the remaining zucchini strips and filling. (You should have 16 enchiladas.) Top the zucchini rolls with the remaining 3/4 cup enchilada sauce and 1/2 cup cheese.

4. Bake until the sauce is bubbling and the cheese is melted, 20 to 25 minutes.

5. Meanwhile, whisk sour cream and milk together in a small bowl. When the enchiladas have finished baking, top with lettuce and cilantro. Drizzle the sour cream mixture over the top.

Prep Time: 25 Minutes

Cook Time: 25 Minutes

Servings: 4

Ingredients

- 1 (2 1/2 to 3 pound) spaghetti squash, cut in half lengthwise and seeds removed
- 3 tablespoons water, divided
- 1 (5 ounce) package baby spinach
- 1 (10 ounce) package frozen artichoke hearts, thawed and chopped
- 4 ounces reduced-fat cream cheese, cubed and softened
- ½ cup grated Parmesan cheese, divided
- ¼ teaspoon salt
- ¼ teaspoon ground pepper
- Crushed red pepper & chopped fresh basil for garnish

Instructions

1. Place squash cut-side down in a microwave-safe dish;
    add 2 tablespoons water. Microwave, uncovered, on
    High until tender, 10 to 15 minutes. (Alternatively,
    place squash halves cut-side down on a rimmed baking
    sheet. Bake at 400 degrees F until tender, 40 to 50
    minutes.)

2. Meanwhile, combine spinach and the remaining 1
    tablespoon water in a large skillet over medium heat.
    Cook, stirring occasionally, until wilted, 3 to 5 minutes.
    Drain and transfer to a large bowl.

3. Position rack in upper third of oven; preheat broiler.

4. Use a fork to scrape the squash from the shells into the
    bowl. Place the shells on a baking sheet. Stir artichoke
    hearts, cream cheese, 1/4 cup Parmesan, salt and
    pepper into the squash mixture. Divide it between the
    squash shells and top with the remaining 1/4 cup
    Parmesan. Broil until the cheese is golden brown,
    about 3 minutes. Sprinkle with crushed red pepper and
    basil, if desired.

Prep Time: 20 Minutes

Cook Time: 20 Minutes

Servings: 4

Ingredients

- 8 ounces whole-wheat rotini
- 1 (5 ounce) package baby spinach, roughly chopped
- 4 ounces reduced-fat cream cheese, cut into chunks
- ¾ cup reduced-fat milk
- ½ cup grated Parmesan cheese, plus more for garnish, if desired
- 2 teaspoons garlic powder
- ¼ teaspoon ground pepper
- 1 (14 ounce) can artichoke hearts, rinsed, squeezed dry and chopped (see Tip)

Instructions

1. Bring a large saucepan of water to a boil. Cook pasta according to package directions. Drain.

2. Combine spinach and 1 tablespoon water in a large saucepan over medium heat. Cook, stirring occasionally, until just wilted, about 2 minutes. Transfer to a small bowl.

3. Add cream cheese and milk to the pan; whisk until the cream cheese is melted.

4. Add Parmesan, garlic powder and pepper; cook, whisking until thickened and bubbling.

5. Drain as much liquid as possible from the spinach. Stir the drained spinach into the sauce, along with artichokes and the pasta. Cook until warmed through.

Prep Time: 45 Minutes

Cook Time: 45 Minutes

Servings: 4

Ingredients

- 2 tablespoons extra-virgin olive oil, divided
- ¼ cup whole-wheat panko breadcrumbs
- 1 tablespoon plus 1 teaspoon minced garlic, divided
- 1 pound boneless, skinless chicken breast, cut into 1/2-inch pieces
- 1 teaspoon Italian seasoning
- ¼ teaspoon salt
- 3 cups low-sodium chicken broth
- 1 ½ cups crushed tomatoes
- 8 ounces whole-wheat penne
- ½ cup shredded mozzarella cheese
- ¼ cup shredded Parmesan cheese
- ¼ cup chopped fresh basil

Instructions

1. Heat 1 tablespoon oil in a large ovenproof skillet over medium-high heat. Add panko and 1 teaspoon garlic. Cook, stirring, until the panko is golden brown, 1 to 2 minutes. Transfer to a small bowl and set aside. Wipe out the pan.

2. Heat the remaining 1 tablespoon oil in the pan over medium-high heat. Add chicken, Italian seasoning, salt and the remaining 1 tablespoon garlic. Cook, stirring frequently, until the chicken is no longer pink on the outside, about 2 minutes. Add broth, tomatoes and penne. Bring to a boil and cook, uncovered, stirring frequently, until the penne is cooked and the sauce has reduced and thickened, 15 to 20 minutes.

3. Meanwhile, position an oven rack in the upper third of the oven. Preheat the broiler to high. When the pasta is cooked, sprinkle mozzarella over the penne mixture. Place the pan under the broiler; broil until the mozzarella is bubbling and beginning to brown, about 1 minute. Top with the panko mixture, Parmesan and basil.

Prep Time: 20 Minutes

Cook Time: 35 Minutes

Servings: 6

Ingredients

- 1 ½ tablespoons extra-virgin olive oil, plus 1 1/2 teaspoons, divided
- 2 (8 ounce) packages sliced fresh button mushrooms
- 1 cup chopped yellow onion
- 3 tablespoons all-purpose flour
- 2 ½ cups whole milk
- 2 teaspoons chopped fresh tarragon
- ½ teaspoon salt
- ½ cup finely grated Parmesan cheese, divided
- 1 pound fresh asparagus, trimmed and cut into 1 inch pieces
- 1 (8.8 ounce) pouch precooked microwaveable whole-grain brown rice or 1 1/2 cups cooked brown rice
- 2 cups chopped cooked chicken breast
- ¼ cup whole-wheat panko breadcrumbs

Instructions

1. Preheat oven to 375 degrees F. Heat 1 1/2 tablespoons oil in a large cast-iron skillet over medium-high heat. Add mushrooms and onion; cook, stirring often, until the moisture released from the vegetables evaporates and the mushrooms are lightly browned, 9 to 10 minutes. Stir in flour; cook, stirring constantly, for 1 minute. Gradually add milk; cook, stirring constantly, until the liquid thickens, about 2 minutes. Stir in tarragon, salt and 1/4 cup Parmesan until melted. Stir in asparagus, rice and chicken. Remove from heat.

2. Toss panko with the remaining 1 1/2 teaspoons oil and 1/4 cup Parmesan in a small bowl; sprinkle over the chicken mixture. Bake until the mixture is bubbly and the topping is golden, about 15 minutes.

Prep Time: 15 Minutes

Cook Time: 25 Minutes

Servings: 4

Ingredients

- 1 (2 1/2- to 3-pound) spaghetti squash, halved lengthwise and seeded
- 1 tablespoon extra-virgin olive oil
- 1 bunch broccolini, chopped
- 4 cloves garlic, minced
- ¼ teaspoon crushed red pepper (optional)
- 2 tablespoons water
- 1 cup shredded part-skim mozzarella cheese, divided
- ¼ cup shredded Parmesan cheese, divided
- ¾ teaspoon Italian seasoning
- ½ teaspoon salt
- ¼ teaspoon ground pepper

Instructions

1. Position racks in upper and lower thirds of oven; preheat to 450 degrees F.

2. Place squash cut-side down in a microwave-safe dish; add 2 tablespoons water. Microwave, uncovered, on High until the flesh is tender, about 10 minutes. (Alternatively, place squash halves cut-side down on a rimmed baking sheet. Bake in a 400 degrees F oven until the squash is tender, 40 to 50 minutes.)

3. Meanwhile, heat oil in a large skillet over medium heat. Add broccolini, garlic and red pepper (if using); cook, stirring frequently, for 2 minutes. Add water and cook, stirring, until the broccolini is tender, 3 to 5 minutes more. Transfer to a large bowl.

4. Use a fork to scrape the squash from the shells into the bowl. Place the shells in a broiler-safe baking pan or on a baking sheet. Stir 3/4 cup mozzarella, 2 tablespoons Parmesan, Italian seasoning, salt and pepper into the squash mixture. Divide it between the shells; top with the remaining 1/4 cup mozzarella and 2 tablespoons Parmesan.

5. Bake on the lower rack for 10 minutes. Move to the upper rack, turn the broiler to high and broil, watching

carefully, until the cheese starts to brown, about 2 minutes.

21. Bone-Building Nourish Bowls

Prep Time: 5 Minutes

Cook Time: 10 Minutes

Servings: 1

Ingredients

- 1 cup spinach
- 2 tbsp carrot grated
- 2 cups brown rice
- 1 egg
- 2 tbsp cheese grated
- 2.5 ounces avocado (half an avocado)
- 1 tbsp olive oil extra virgin
- 1/2 cup blueberries
- 1 tbsp sesame seeds
- 1 tsp pesto to top
- 1/2 fresh squeezed lemon

Instructions

1. Start by prepping your ingredients!

2. Cook your brown rice as per package instructions.

3. Place your egg in a pot and add cold water until the whole egg is covered and there's an additional 1 inch of water on top. Bring to a boil over medium-high heat, then cover. Remove from heat and set aside for 8 to 10 minutes. Drain and place in a bowl of cold water to cool. Once cool, you can peel your egg.

4. Wash all your fruits and veggies. Grate your carrots and cheese, and slice your avocado.

5. Once all your ingredients are prepped, it's time to assemble your bowl. Start by placing your rice at the bottom of the bowl. Then, make it look pretty by arranging the rest of your ingredients separately on top— like I do in the video!

6. Squeeze half a lemon over your bowl and finish with a drizzle of olive oil!

Prep Time: 5 Minutes

Cook Time: 15 Minutes

Servings: 1

Ingredients

- 1 cup tahini
- 1/2 tsp cinnamon
- 1/2 cup coconut sugar
- 2 Tbs ground chia (mixed with 1/3 c water) OR 1 egg
- 1 cup rolled oats
- 1 cup coconut flakes
- 1/4 cup raisins
- 1/4 cup cacao nibs
- 1/4 cup chocolate chips
- 1/3 cup walnuts, chopped
- pinch sea salt

Instructions

1. Pre-heat oven to 350. In a large bowl, mix tahini, chia mixture (or egg), cinnamon, coconut sugar, pinch sea

salt until well combined, then mix remaining ingredients. You might want to get in there with your hands to ensure it's well combined and dough-like consistency is formed.

2. Roll into gold-size balls in your hands, then press flat on cookie sheet lined with parchment paper or greased with coconut oil. Smooth top and form into rounds. Bake until golden, about 20 minutes. Let cool completely before eating.

Prep Time: 20 Minutes

Cook Time: 30 Minutes

Servings: 4

Ingredients

- 1 cup (250 mL) milk
- 1/2 cup (125 mL) water
- 3/4 tsp. (3 mL) dried oregano
- 1/4 tsp (1 mL) salt
- 1/4 tsp (1 mL) pepper
- 1cup (250 mL) quinoa, rinsed
- 1 lemon, grated zest
- 2 tbsp (30 mL) lemon juice
- 1 yellow sweet pepper, chopped
- 1 English cucumber, chopped
- 1/2 cup (125 mL) red onion, diced
- 1cup (250 mL) canned red beans, drained, rinsed
- 1 cup (250 mL) Feta cheese, diced
- 1 grilled chicken, slice

Instructions

Dinner: Quinoa Greek Salad with Grilled Chicken

1. In a deep saucepan, combine milk, water, oregano, salt and pepper. Bring to boil over medium heat. Stir in quinoa. Reduce heat to low, cover and simmer for 20 minutes. Let stand covered 5 minutes. Transfer to bowl.

2. Stir in lemon zest with fork; let cool. Stir in remaining ingredients. Serve on a plate with grilled chicken. (Serve or refrigerate up to 1 day.)

Tip: Next time you're cooking or baking, try using milk instead of water. Milk products are one of the most under-consumed food groups by adults. Studies show that the nutrients in milk can help you achieve and maintain a healthy weight; the protein in milk products helps build muscle mass and keeps you feeling fuller for longer.

Prep Time: 20 Minutes

Cook Time: 40 Minutes

Servings: 4

Ingredients

- 1 large head broccoli, cut into florets, blanched or steamed, drained well
- 3 tbsp mayonnaise
- Juice of 1 lemon
- 1/4 cup grated Parmesan cheese
- 3 tbsp olive oil
- 1 tbsp Dijon mustard
- 1 tsp Worcestershire sauce
- 2 garlic cloves, minced
- To taste salt and freshly ground pepper
- 2 slices pancetta or bacon, cooked and chopped

For garnishing Parmesan cheese

Instructions

1. Combine mayonnaise, lemon juice, Parmesan, olive oil, Dijon mustard, Worcestershire sauce, garlic, and salt and pepper.
2. Add broccoli and toss to combine. Finish with pancetta and freshly grated Parmesan, or use a vegetable peeler to garnish with shards of Parmesan cheese.

Prep Time: 15 Minutes

Cook Time: 30 Minutes

Servings: 4

Ingredients

- 1 1/3 cups (325 mL) water
- 1/3 cup (75 mL) buckwheat groats
- 1/3 cup (75 mL) quinoa seeds
- 1/2 cup (125 mL) walnuts
- 3 cups (750 mL) broccoli pieces, broccoli florets and peeled diced stalk
- 1/3 cup (75 mL) dried sweetened cranberries
- 1/3 cup (75 mL) finely diced red onion
- 1/4 cup (60 mL) liquid honey or pure maple syrup
- 1/4 cup (60 mL) red wine vinegar
- 2 tbsp (30 mL) olive or walnut oil
- 1/2 tsp (2 mL) minced garlic
- pinch salt, optional

Instructions

1. Combine the water, buckwheat and quinoa in a small saucepan and bring to a boil. Reduce to a simmer, cover and cooks for 15 minutes. Remove from the heat, fluff with a fork and cool completely.

2. Heat a saute pan on medium heat and place the walnuts in the pan. Stir frequently until the walnuts are fragrant and toasted. Remove from the heat, cool slightly and coarsely chop. Set aside.

3. Place completely cooked grains, broccoli, walnuts, cranberries and red onion in a large bowl. Whisk together the honey, vinegar, oil, garlic and salt (if using). Toss with the vegetable mixture and serve.

Prep Time: 20 Minutes

Cook Time: 30 Minutes

Servings: 4

Ingredients

- 2-3 bunches broccolini
- 1 cup red pearl onions
- 1 tablespoon olive oil
- 1 tablespoon butter
- to taste salt and pepper
- Trim broccolini ends.

Instructions

1. Blanch broccolini for 30 seconds to 1 minute, drain.
2. Blanch pearl onions for 30 seconds to one minute until skins start to come off.
3. Drain, peel and halve pearl onions.
4. Add to hot pan with butter and olive oil.
5. Toss around for a few minutes.
6. Season with salt and pepper.

7. Transfer to serving platter.

Prep Time: 20 Minutes

Cook Time: 30 Minutes

Servings: 4

Ingredients

- 2 whole acorn squash, small
- 2 tbsp coconut oil
- 1/4 cup onion, diced
- to taste sea salt
- to taste pepper
- 2 cups cooked quinoa
- 1 1/2 cups fresh spinach, chopped
- 1/4 cup dried apricots, chopped
- 1/4 cup dried cranberries
- 1/3 cup pecans, toasted and chopped
- 1/2 cup pomegranate seeds
- 1/4 cup flat-leaf parsley, chopped
- 1/2 tsp ground cinnamon
- 2 tbsp extra virgin olive oil
- 1 tbsp lemon juice
- 2 tsp maple syrup

Instructions

1. Cut the acorn squash in half, scoop out the seeds, and then place the halves cut-side down on a baking sheet, greased with 1 tablespoon of coconut oil. Roast until soft (about 30 minutes).

2. Heat 1 tablespoon of coconut oil in a large skillet over medium heat. Add the onions and a pinch of salt and pepper and cook, stirring, until golden (about 15 minutes). Stir in cooked quinoa and add spinach.

3. Remove from heat and cover, just until the spinach wilts (about a minute or two). Add remaining ingredients to the skillet and stir to blend.

4. Remove squash from the oven. Scoop out part of the flesh, chop and then stir into the quinoa blend.

5. Use the halved squash as bowls for the salad.

Prep Time: 20 Minutes

Cook Time: 30 Minutes

Servings: 4

Ingredients

- 2 cups quinoa
- 4 ½ cups water
- ¾ tsp salt plus more for boiling water
- 3 tbsp extra-virgin olive oil
- 1 ½ tbsp fresh lemon juice
- 1 19oz can black beans, drained and rinsed well
- 1 red pepper, seeded and finely diced
- ½ cup feta cheese, chopped into a small dice
- 2 scallions, very finely chopped
- ½ cup fresh parsley, chopped

Instructions

1. Bring a large pot of salted water to boil. Add rinsed quinoa and cook, stirring occasionally for 8-10 minutes, or until grains have expanded and tails have popped out. Drain

through a fine mesh sieve under running water, then allow to sit for 5 minutes.

2. Spread cooked quinoa out onto a paper towel-lined sheet pan to dry for 20 minutes. Transfer to a bowl. Season with salt, olive oil, lemon juice, scallion and parsley and mix well. Add black beans, peppers and feta and toss gently to combine. Taste and adjust seasoning as necessary.

Prep Time: 5 Minutes

Cook Time: 20 Minutes

Servings: 1

Ingredients

- 1 cup (250 mL) milk
- 1/2 cup (125 mL) water
- 3/4 tsp (3 mL) dried oregano
- 1/4 tsp (1 mL) salt
- 1/4 tsp (1 mL) pepper
- 1cup (250 mL) quinoa, rinsed
- 1 lemon, grated zest
- 2 tbsp (30 mL) lemon juice
- 1 yellow sweet pepper, chopped
- 1 English cucumber, chopped
- 1/2 cup (125 mL) red onion , diced
- 1cup (250 mL) canned red beans, drained, rinsed
- 1 cup (250 mL) Feta cheese , diced
- 1 grilled chicken, slice

Instructions

Dinner: Quinoa Greek Salad with Grilled Chicken

1. In a deep saucepan, combine milk, water, oregano, salt and pepper. Bring to boil over medium heat. Stir in quinoa. Reduce heat to low, cover and simmer for 20 minutes. Let stand covered 5 minutes. Transfer to bowl.

2. Stir in lemon zest with fork; let cool. Stir in remaining ingredients. Serve on a plate with grilled chicken.(Serve or refrigerate up to 1 day.)

Prep Time: 00 Minutes

Cook Time: 00 Minutes

Servings: 2

Ingredients

- ½ batch farinata batter
- ¼ cup olive oil plus 2 tbsp
- Freshly ground pepper
- 8 thin slices prosciutto
- 1 clove garlic, minced
- ½ yellow cooking onion, thinly sliced
- ½ bunch kale, stemmed and leaves chopped into 1-inch pieces
- ½ tsp kosher salt
- Juice of 1 lemon

Instructions

1. Make farinata according to recipe, and cut into quarters when it comes out of the oven.

2. In a separate sauté pan, heat 2 tbsp olive oil on medium high heat. Add onion and sauté for 2 minute. Add garlic and sauté for another minute, being careful not to brown.

3. Add kale and season with salt and pepper. Toss to coat kale in onion garlic mixture and cook for 3-5 minutes, or until kale is wilted but still bright green. Squeeze lemon juice over kale off the heat.

4. To plate, lay 2 slices of prosciutto down on one quartered wedge of farinata and top with a pile of kale.